The Need to Know Nutrition and Healthy Eating

The Perfect Starter To Eating Well

Or

How To Eat The Right Foods, Stay In Shape And Stick To A Healthy Diet

TIM SHAW BSc MSc

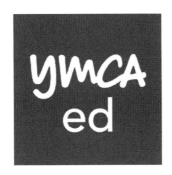

Discover more books and ebooks of interest to you and find out about the range of work we do at the forefront of health, fitness and wellbeing.

www.centralymcaguides.com

Published by Central YMCA Trading Ltd (trading as YMCAed).
Registered Company No. 3667206.

Central YMCA is the world's founding YMCA. Established in 1844 in Central London, it was the first YMCA to open its doors and, in so doing, launched a movement that has now grown to become the world's biggest youth organisation. Today, Central YMCA is the UK's leading health, fitness and wellbeing charity, committed to helping people from all walks of life – and particularly the young and those with a specific need – to live happier, healthier and more fulfilled lives.

ISBN: 1481294784
ISBN-13: 978-1481294782

CONTENTS

ABOUT THE AUTHOR

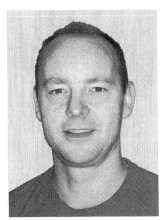 Hello and thanks for reading this book.

I am an experienced instructor in the health and fitness industry, specialising in teaching the principles of exercise, nutrition and healthy eating to gym instructors and personal trainers. I am also involved in teaching fitness for disabled clients and training for older adults.

I have worked for London Central YMCA as a tutor in health and fitness for over 20 years. Prior to that I studied engineering and have a BSc in technology and an MSc in robotics.

My interest in nutrition first began back in the 1980s and over the past three decades I have tried most diets and food fads for myself, ultimately concluding that they are largely unnecessary and that the best nutrition is actually achieved by following simple guidelines and eating the right balance of healthy foods.

I hope you enjoy the book.

Tim

INTRODUCTION

First things first, this isn't a diet book; it's a simple guide to healthy eating.

In other words, the following pages will not advise you to follow any radical changes in your eating habits. Instead, you will learn the basics of good nutrition and the many benefits that can result.

Indeed, there is now a wealth of irrefutable evidence to suggest that good diet has a range of positive health consequences. Furthermore, there is also reasonable consensus amongst nutritionists as to what a 'good diet' for most people actually is. This book will therefore introduce you to some simple guidelines which, if you decide to follow them and commit to a positive new eating habit, will help you to:

- control your body weight and lose excess fat without dieting
- have more energy, better mood and concentration
- have a stronger immune system to fight infection
- keep your blood pressure and blood cholesterol levels within healthy ranges
- have a healthier heart and circulatory system with less chance of a heart attack or stroke
- reduce your risk of getting certain forms of cancer
- have a better sex life and improved fertility
- live longer and lead a more active life.

There are lots more benefits, but that's a long enough list for now.

The advice you're about to read is designed to be practical more than theoretical. Useful information has been condensed and divided into easy bite size form, so you can dip in and out when convenient, or use it for quick reference when shopping or buying your lunch.

Expect a long-term healthy eating plan, not a short-term fix. Also, expect to contribute a little time and discipline yourself.

There are many diet fads you can follow that will promise quick weight loss, but they all involve major dietary changes and can create a range of health problems as a result, including low energy levels, depression, unhealthy changes to hormone levels, reduced vitamin and mineral status, lowered metabolism, and so on.

Unless the change in your eating habit is sustainable, you will, at some point, return to your old ways and your original problems of poor health and weight gain will return. So, while we won't be telling you to radically change what you eat, you will need to commit to eating healthily in the long term.

Read on to find out how.

1

A BALANCED, HEALTHY DIET

The human body remains in good health and functions most efficiently if it obtains the food it needs in the right quantities and with the correct balance.

The easiest way to ensure an optimum balance of nutrients is to divide foods into six main groups and then, over a normal day's eating, aim to consume the recommended number of portions of each group. The table below outlines commonly endorsed portion recommendations.

Food Group	Recommended portions per day
Complex carbohydrates	6 - 11
Fruit and vegetables	5 - 9
Protein-rich foods	2 - 3
Dairy	2 - 3
Healthy fats	2 - 3
Foods high in unhealthy fats and refined sugar	0 – 1 (eat sparingly)

(www.dh.gov.uk, 2012) (www.choosemyplate.gov, 2012) (www.hsph.harvard.edu, 2012) (Bean, 2003)

Many authorities use a picture of a food plate to represent healthy proportions of these food groups. Complex carbohydrates and fruit and vegetables take up the largest segments of the plate, followed by smaller segments of protein-rich foods, dairy foods and healthy fats. The thinnest wedge is reserved for foods high in unhealthy fats and refined sugar. Note that National Guidelines in the UK have been slightly adapted here, with the addition of recommended portion numbers, and an allowance given for healthy fats.

It isn't realistic to get this balance at every single meal or snack. Rather, you should try to get the balance right on *most* days. If this is hard because of work, study, travel or family commitments, you might find it easier to achieve a healthy balance over a longer timeframe of a whole week. This gives you some flexibility for socialising and having the occasional lapse.

WHAT IS A PORTION?

You can use the following examples as a guide to portion sizes for each food group.

Although there are only a few foods listed here, they should be enough for you to estimate portions for most other foods you eat – simply look for the most similar item:

Complex carbohydrates: 1 slice of bread, 1 small bread roll, 1 potato, ½ cup of cooked rice or pasta, 30g (just over 1oz) breakfast cereal, etc.

Fruit and vegetables: 1 medium fruit (apple, orange, banana, etc.), handful of berries or grapes, one 125ml (5fl oz) glass of fruit juice or smoothie, 1 small bowl of salad, ½ cup of cooked vegetables.

Protein-rich foods: Meat, fish, chicken, tofu (size of a deck of cards), 1 egg, ½ cup of cooked beans or pulses, etc.

Dairy: One 200ml (⅓ pint) glass of milk, 1 small carton of yoghurt, 40g (nearly 2oz) cheese (size of a small matchbox).

Healthy fats: 2 teaspoons of olive oil, oily fish (size of a deck of cards), ½ an avocado, 2 tablespoons of nuts or seeds, etc.

Foods high in unhealthy fats and refined sugar: 1 biscuit, 1 slice of cake, 1 can of soft drink, 25g (1oz) bag of crisps, 1 small bowl of chocolate pudding, 125ml glass fruit juice or smoothie (if you have more than 1 per day), etc.

Later in the book we will look at each of the food groups in more detail to find out what they contribute to a healthy diet and why we are advised to eat them in these proportions.

HOW CAN I KEEP TRACK OF WHAT I EAT?

A practical idea is to use a table to record the portions of each food group you eat on a daily basis. The table is blank at the start of the day, and you simply add a mark whenever you consume a portion of that particular food group. At the end of the day you can total each column to see how close you are to the recommended portions. It may look something like this:

Foods group	Complex carbohydrates	Fruit and vegetables	Protein-rich foods	Dairy	Healthy fats	Foods high in unhealthy fats and refined sugar
Portions eaten	||||| ||| Total = 8	|| Total = 2	||| Total = 3	||| Total = 3		 Total = 1	||||| || Total = 7
Portions recommended	6 - 11	5 - 9	2 - 3	2 - 3	2 - 3	0 - 1

Better still, use this method to keep track of what you eat over several days and then average your portions to give a more complete picture of your diet.

In this example the portions of complex carbohydrates, protein-rich foods and dairy are all *about* right. Healthy fats are lower than recommended. Most significantly, however, the intake of fruit and vegetables clearly needs to increase, and the quantity of foods high in processed fats and sugars is much too high. So it is easy to identify how eating can be improved the very next day, and improvements can be made gradually. In this case, a good start would be to decline one of the fatty, sugary snacks and replace it with some fruit instead.

This type of analysis is easy, takes little time, and yields useful, practical results. If you would like a more in-depth analysis that counts calories, calculates exact percentages of fats, proteins and carbohydrates, and evaluates intake of important vitamins and minerals, then there are various websites and smartphone apps that can help in this complex task.

2

HOW MUCH TO EAT

In this section we will answer a few basic questions about energy, metabolism and how much to eat.

Your body requires energy from food to perform basic metabolic functions of living, and for daily activity and exercise. Eating the correct amount of food to give us energy is therefore essential for maintaining a healthy body weight and for feeling energetic enough for daily activities.

If you don't eat enough food to supply all the energy you need, then inevitably you will feel tired, you will lack concentration, you may feel depressed and eventually your health will suffer. You will also lose weight, but this needs to be managed carefully so that fat is shed steadily over weeks and months, without suffering all the unhealthy consequences of not eating enough food.

On the other hand, if you eat too much food, then you may suffer digestive discomfort, and the excess of energy you have consumed will be stored as body fat. In a modern developed country, where high calorie foods containing lots of fat and sugar are widely available, it is very easy to eat too much food.

Our need for food intake to match our energy expenditure is neatly illustrated using these energy balance equations:

Energy in = energy out (results in weight maintenance)
Energy in > energy out (results in weight gain)
Energy in < energy out (results in weight loss)

Energy is measured in kilocalories, which is commonly written on food packaging as kcal. However, we usually just say 'calories' for convenience.

HOW MANY CALORIES SHOULD I EAT EACH DAY?

It follows that, in order to know how many calories to eat each day (energy in), we first have to know how many calories we expend (energy out). If the two are equal then your needs will be met and you will maintain a healthy weight.

'Energy out' depends on two main factors: basal metabolic rate and activity.

1. Basal metabolic rate (BMR): this is the sum of all your metabolic processes – things like keeping your heart beating, breathing, creating body heat and brain function.

You can estimate your basal metabolic rate using the simple formula:

BMR = body weight (kg) x 25

For example:

- If you weigh 60kg your BMR is approximately: 60 x 25 = 1500kcal
- If you weigh 80kg your BMR is approximately: 80 x 25 = 2000kcal

The larger your body, the higher your BMR. This is an important point to remember if you want to increase your metabolic rate.

2. Activity: This can be estimated using a physical activity factor (PAF) with which to multiply the BMR:

Inactive: PAF = 1.2 (desk job, drive everywhere or take public transport, negligible exercise or active pastimes)

Moderately active: PAF = 1.5 (moderately active job involving standing, walking, etc. Regular 3 x weekly gym visits or playing social sports)

Very active: PAF = 1.8 (very active job involving lifting and carrying, etc. Regular 5 x weekly gym visits with intense, longer duration training sessions or playing intense, competitive sports)

To calculate **total daily energy expenditure**, the formula is **BMR x PAF**. For example:

- If you weigh 60kg and you are inactive, your daily total is: 1500 x 1.2 = 1800kcal
- If you weigh 80kg and you are very active, your daily total is: 2000 x 1.8 = 3600kcal

In other words, if you are the 60kg person, you need to eat about 1800kcal per day to maintain weight. If the 80kg person is closer to you, you need about 3600kcal per day, which is considerably more, but is justified by your larger body and much higher activity level.

If you want to keep a detailed record of what you eat and how many calories you consume, then this calculation is a useful guide to how much you should eat. However, it's not really necessary. The food plate and portion numbers work just as well.

HOW DO CALORIES RELATE TO THE FOOD PLATE?

Following the portion numbers from the food plate equates closely to a healthy calorie intake. If you are closer to the 1800kcal per day example we quoted above, this would be supplied by the lower portion numbers (6 of complex carbohydrates, 5 of fruit and vegetables, 2 of protein-rich foods, etc.). If you need closer to 3600kcal per day, this will be met by the higher portion numbers (11 of complex carbs, 9 of fruit and veg, 3 of protein-rich foods, etc.). If these portion numbers still don't meet your needs, then you can eat more; just use the plate as a guide to keeping the proportions healthy.

HOW CAN I INCREASE MY ENERGY EXPENDITURE?

It follows from the energy calculation that there are two possible ways of increasing energy expenditure:

1. Increase metabolism
2. Increase activity

Basal metabolism can be increased within certain limits by increasing the amount of healthy lean tissue you have; in other words, by increasing how much muscle you have. The easiest way to do this in a structured way is to use resistance training.

Activity can be increased in a variety of ways: by active daily living such as walking, gardening and housework. Pastimes such as golf or rambling increase activity levels in a relaxed and pleasurable way. Playing sports or going to the gym are other possibilities. However, this book is primarily about healthy eating, so we won't dwell too long on exercise.

IS THERE SUCH A THING AS A NATURALLY SLOW OR FAST METABOLISM?

You will frequently hear some people say they are overweight because they have a 'naturally slow metabolism' or others say they can eat what they want and not put on weight because they have a 'fast metabolism'. Although it is tempting to believe this idea and it may *appear* to be the case, controlled studies have failed to find these radically 'slow' or 'fast' metabolisers. Basal metabolic rate is not decided by some pre-set control; instead it depends mainly on your body weight.

Science does offer an alternative explanation for apparent differences between people's ability to control body weight. Careful observations reveal that there are big variations in spontaneous activity levels between individuals. Those who tend towards obesity are naturally more sedentary, whilst those who tend towards thinness are more active and 'always on the go'. This is possibly hard wired in the genes (a natural 'set point' for how active you are) and also influenced by lifestyle in early childhood, where obesity leads to inactivity as the child gets older (www.earlybirddiabetes.org 2012).

3

WHEN TO EAT

A regular meal structure is essential to healthy eating. There are two main reasons for this. The first is to give an even supply of energy and nutrients to your body throughout the day. The second is to control hunger. A practical meal plan is to have three balanced main meals – breakfast, lunch and dinner – with two or three healthy snacks in between to moderate hunger and elevate mood and energy levels.

Breakfast is particularly important in the day's eating plan, yet it can be very tempting to miss breakfast altogether, either as a way to lose weight, or because you just don't have time. However, consider this: if you eat an evening meal at 8pm one day, then skip breakfast the next morning and don't eat again until lunch time, that's a total of 17 hours out of 24 where you are fasting and have no energy or nutrient intake.

You might argue that this is a good way to cut out calories and lose weight, but there are other factors to consider. Your mood, concentration and energy levels will suffer throughout the morning, particularly around 10.30 – 11am when blood sugar levels tend to hit a natural low.

More importantly, when you eat again at lunch time you are much more likely to binge on high fat and high sugar foods, taking in all of the calories you would have done anyway had you eaten breakfast. Relatively recent research has identified certain 'hunger hormones' released by your stomach and fat cells in response to several hours of fasting. The longer you fast, the higher the level of these hunger hormones, making you crave calorie-dense fats and sugars.

DOES IT MATTER IF I EAT MY MAIN MEAL IN THE EVENING?

You will often hear people advising you not to eat your main meal in the evening, or 'no carbs after 6pm' and so on. However, the evidence for these arbitrary rules is limited. The usual justification for this advice is that, if several hours of sleep follow a big meal, you will store all the calories you have just eaten as fat. Better to eat those calories in the morning and burn them up during the day so your body doesn't store them.

However, the counter argument is that so long as your total day's calories don't exceed your needs, things will even out over a longer timeframe of a few days; anything stored one night is simply used the next day.

Also, it makes a lot of sense for nutrients to be available to your body as it recovers and repairs overnight. So there is nothing inherently wrong with eating healthy food at this time of the day. In fact, eating a main meal in the evening is so universal and inherent to social convention that simply to say 'don't do this' is unrealistic. It is possible that eating at the end of the day (after all that hunting and gathering) is deeply rooted in our circadian rhythms (Foster & Kreitzman, 2005).

There is another factor to consider here. Whilst a balanced evening meal is a fine and pleasurable thing, you should resist the temptation to continue snacking afterwards. It is so easy to lapse and keep visiting the kitchen for some potato nibbles, corn chips, ice cream plus a glass or two of wine. The time of day is not the pivotal factor here; it is more that you feel tired, bored or stressed and you use your fridge full of treats to help relax and unwind.

4

COMPLEX CARBOHYDRATES

We should aim to eat 6 to 11 portions per day.

Examples of portions include: 1 slice of bread, 1 small bread roll, 1 potato, ½ cup of cooked rice or pasta, 30g (just over 1oz) breakfast cereal.

Complex carbohydrates form one of the largest segments of the healthy eating plate and should be a significant part of our daily eating because they are such a good source of energy, fibre, vitamins and minerals. They also supply significant protein to the diet and they are relatively inexpensive when compared to meat, poultry, fish and dairy foods. However, despite all of these positive points, carbohydrates continue to suffer from bad press because of the popularity of low-carb diets and the notion that 'carbs make you fat'.

Experience tells us that low-carb diets can definitely result in rapid weight loss. However, before you are tempted to try this approach, consider some of the wider aspects of your health that may be affected. Without carbs in the diet you are likely to suffer from a serious lack of energy, depressed mood and lower concentration. You will also have a lower fibre intake due to lack of whole grains, which will affect your bowel function. Vitamin and mineral intake are likely to be compromised too. Your body still needs energy to function and without carbs it must obtain this from the fats and proteins you eat. Metabolism of fats in the absence of enough carbohydrates leads to a state called 'ketosis'. The most noticeable sign of ketosis is a distinctive smell to the breath.

Eliminating carbohydrates from your diet is not a sensible long-term plan. Instead *'good carbs, not no carbs'* should be your rule.

WHAT TYPE OF COMPLEX CARBS SHOULD I EAT?

You should choose unrefined complex carbohydrates where possible in preference to refined products. This is because unrefined carbs include the vitamins, minerals and fibre that your body needs. They take time to digest, releasing their energy relatively slowly, satisfying your appetite for longer. Slow release of energy also makes it harder to store calories as fat. Examples of unrefined carbs include wholemeal bread, wholegrain rice and whole wheat pasta. Also consider alternatives to wheat-based, unrefined carbohydrates, e.g. oats, barley and rye.

Refined carbs supply the energy component, but they don't necessarily have the vitamins, minerals and fibre of the unrefined carbs. Their refined state means your gut digests them and releases their energy more quickly, so although you satisfy your hunger rapidly you will feel hungry again soon. Quick energy release also makes it more likely that calories will be stored as fat. Examples of refined complex carbs include white bread, white rice and regular pasta.

A wise plan is to base meals and snacks primarily on unrefined complex carbohydrates to ensure you obtain all of the nutrition in a complete package to keep you feeling fuller for longer.

WHY IS FIBRE IMPORTANT?

Fibre is the 'roughage' part of unrefined complex carbs. Other plant foods like pulses, fruit and vegetables are also excellent sources of fibre. There are two main types of fibre and most foods contain a mixture of both.

Insoluble fibre cannot be digested by your body. It is resilient to the acid and digestive juices in the stomach and remains largely intact when passing through the intestines. In other words, it leaves your body in much the same form as it went in (think of sweet corn...). Insoluble fibre is not absorbed from the digestive tract into the blood and is therefore not an essential nutrient, strictly speaking. However, it does have important health benefits: it adds bulk to the food you eat, helping it to move through the gut more easily. In particular, it keeps your bowels healthy, helping to prevent constipation.

Soluble fibre can be digested by your body. It may help to reduce the amount of LDL (bad) cholesterol in your blood. Porridge oats, beans, lentils and many fruits are all good sources of soluble fibre.

Foods that are high in both types of fibre take longer to leave your stomach and will keep you feeling fuller for longer, which can be useful if you are trying to lose weight.

Typical fibre intake per day is around 14g. Health guidelines suggest you should be aiming to eat at least 18g, along with plenty of fluids (www.nhs.uk 2012). However, there is no need to check grams on food labels. Fibre intake is naturally taken care of if you eat the recommended portions of unrefined carbohydrates, fruit and vegetables. It is unnecessary to eat any special foods or add fibre supplements, such as bran, to your diet. In fact, too much fibre can cause bloating, wind, abdominal discomfort and reduced nutrient absorption.

WHAT IS GI?

GI stands for glycaemic index. It is a way of measuring how quickly carbohydrates are digested and raise your blood sugar level. Glucose is used as the reference food (GI = 100) and then other foods are compared to this reference point and given a number on a 1 to 100 scale.

High GI carbs such as a breakfast cereal (GI = 80+) will raise blood sugar significantly within minutes of ingestion. Lower GI carbs such as those found in apples (GI = 38) or porridge (GI = 42) take much longer to have any measurable effect on blood sugar. This matters because a quick peak in blood sugar from high GI carbs stimulates your pancreas to release a large amount of insulin which in turn causes blood sugar to decrease quickly as it transports sugar into the cells. This 'trough' in blood sugar makes you feel tired, irritable, unable to concentrate and hungry (low blood sugar is a powerful hunger signal for the brain).

A low GI carb gives a slower rise in blood sugar and so avoids the large release of insulin and therefore avoids the reactive low blood sugar that follows. You feel more energetic, less irritable, you are able to concentrate and you feel fuller for longer. Low GI foods may play a role in helping to prevent non-insulin dependent diabetes. Research has shown that lower GI diets have also been associated with a lower incidence of heart disease (www.diabetes.org.uk 2012). So the rule is to eat low GI carbs when you can.

How can you tell if carbs are high GI or low GI?

There is a general belief that sugary carbs are fast acting high GI and starchy complex carbs are slow acting and low GI, but this is not the case and the truth is much more complicated.

For example, the carbohydrate in apples is all sugar and yet they are low GI. This is because the sugar in apples is mainly in the form of fructose (or fruit sugar) which your body takes much longer to digest than glucose.

White bread, which contains mainly complex carbohydrates, has a high GI. It happens that the intense processing involved in the production of a modern white loaf makes the starch particles very easy for your body to break down and utilise. Baked potatoes actually have a higher GI than boiled potatoes (it's to do with the cooking process).

With so many factors contributing to GI, you will probably be thinking, 'Do I have to consult a GI reference table every time I eat carbs?' Well you could do this if you have the time, but a simpler way is just to follow the unrefined rule. Not only do unrefined carbs give us vitamins, minerals and fibre but they also tend to be lower GI as well.

One final point about GI. The number only applies to a portion of carbs eaten in isolation. As soon as fats and proteins are combined with the carbs, then digestion and the blood sugar spike are slowed significantly. For example, high GI white bread combined with butter, cheese and pickle to make a tasty sandwich, results in a lower GI meal. This leads to the final point about complex carbs: eat them as part of a balanced meal or snack that also contains proteins and healthy fats.

5

FRUITS AND VEGETABLES

We should aim to eat between 5 and 9 portions per day.

Examples of portions include: 1 medium fruit (apple, orange, banana, etc.), one 125ml (5fl oz) glass fruit juice or smoothie, a handful of berries or grapes, 1 small bowl of salad, ½ cup of cooked vegetables.

We are advised to eat a lot of fruit and veg because they are packed with important vitamins (especially vitamin C) and minerals (particularly potassium and magnesium), they are high in water content, bulk and fibre and they are usually low in fat. Note that there are some exceptions to the low fat rule, such as avocados and olives, but even then they count as 'healthy fats'. In addition, fruit and veg contain antioxidant phytochemicals that have further health benefits.

WHAT ARE ANTIOXIDANTS?

Antioxidants are substances found in food that help to prevent cellular damage from oxygen free radicals. Free radicals are inevitable by-products of respiration and oxygen use in the body. They are very unstable molecules and can damage cells unless they are neutralised, or 'quenched', by antioxidants. The most effective antioxidants from food are vitamin C from fresh fruit and vegetables, vitamin E from wheat germ, fruit, nuts, cereals, etc. and a number of phytochemicals.

WHAT ARE PHYTOCHEMICALS?

Phytochemicals are substances found in plants that can have a beneficial effect on our health ('phyto' is Greek for 'plant'). You may have heard results of research saying that, among other foods, red wine, grapes, berries, garlic, onions, tea, tomatoes and broccoli are all good for us. This advice is usually based on phytochemicals they contain, such as carotenoids and flavanoids. Although phytochemicals are not counted as essential nutrients, many of them appear to have a significant protective effect against the development of heart disease and cancer. This is possibly why there is a strong link between eating lots of plant foods and a lowered risk of suffering from these health problems.

We have all heard of the 'five a day' recommendation, yet many of us still find it hard to eat enough to meet this simple guideline. This is because they can require more effort and preparation than convenience foods like crisps, flapjacks and chocolate bars. They also have less immediate appeal to our taste buds. Most people, given the choice between an apple and a bar of chocolate, will choose the chocolate.

HOW CAN I INCREASE MY FRUIT AND VEG INTAKE?

Here are a few practical ways you can try to increase your daily portions of fruit and veg that don't take a lot of time or effort:

- 125ml of fruit juice or smoothie counts as a portion. So pour yourself a glass of orange juice each morning, or have one small carton from the supermarket with lunch (but more than one fruit juice and it starts to count as sugar intake).
- Add a chopped banana or handful of berries to your breakfast cereal.
- Make a habit of having a side salad with lunch or dinner.

Blend vegetables into a soup. This is a useful way to include more veg without it being noticed. Ideal for recalcitrant children of all ages.

6

PROTEIN-RICH FOODS

We should aim to eat 2 to 3 portions per day.

Examples of portions include: Meat, fish, chicken, tofu (size of a deck of cards), 1 egg, ½ cup of cooked beans or pulses.

Protein-rich foods are well known as being important for growth and repair of body tissues. However, they have a whole range of other functions too: they support the immune system; they are essential for hormone and enzyme production; and they can also supply significant energy.

WHAT PROTEIN FOODS ARE BEST?

Animal proteins such as meat, fish, poultry and eggs are called 'complete' because they supply all of the amino acids your body needs for growth and repair. Non-animal proteins like beans, lentils, cereals and nuts are 'incomplete' because each is missing some vital amino acids. So in this respect, animal proteins are higher quality than non-animal proteins. An exception to this rule is the soya bean. Soya-based products such as tofu (soya bean curd) or soya milk are considered to be complete proteins because they contain such a good range of amino acids.

However, before planning meals based around chicken, steak, tuna and omelettes, there are other factors to consider. Animal proteins are expensive and often come packaged together with high fat (50% of the calories in a good steak will be from fat. An egg is even higher at around

60% fat). In contrast, most non-animal proteins like beans and lentils are inexpensive and naturally low in fat. In addition, it is easy to improve the quality of these proteins and make them complete simply by combining two or more foods together. For example, baked beans on whole wheat toast combines beans with wheat giving a complete source of protein. A peanut butter sandwich gives a similar result.

WILL I OBTAIN ENOUGH PROTEIN IF I AM VEGETARIAN OR VEGAN?

Concerns about vegetarian eating and lack of protein are generally unfounded, so long as the healthy eating plate is followed and there are sufficient protein-rich foods included. In fact, vegetarian and vegan eating approaches have many positive benefits. They are low in saturated fat, low in salt and high in fibre, vitamins and minerals when compared to meat eaters.

Vegetarians can easily get enough protein from a well-planned diet because there are still complete proteins in milk, cheese, yoghurt, eggs, tofu and soya milk. Then there are the incomplete proteins in beans, pulses, nuts, seeds and cereals which, when eaten in combination, provide more than enough essential amino acids for protein needs to be met. Even if incomplete proteins are eaten at different meals throughout the day, the amino acids are available to the body long enough for the necessary combinations to be formed.

If you are vegan and eat no animal products at all, you will find it a little harder to get sufficient protein. But it is still possible. The main complete protein sources available to you are soya products and the remainder must come from good combinations of plant proteins.

7

DAIRY FOODS

We should aim to eat 2 to 3 portions per day.

Examples of portions include: One 200ml (⅓ pint) glass of milk, 1 small carton of yoghurt, 40g (nearly 2oz) cheese (size of a small matchbox).

Dairy foods such as milk, cheese and yoghurt are a good source of protein. However they are not counted along with other protein foods on the food plate, and instead are given a place of their own. This is because they are a particularly good source of calcium, essential for strong bones and teeth.

One potential problem with consuming dairy foods is their high fat content and therefore their high calories. If the guideline of 2 to 3 portions per day is followed, then this shouldn't be a problem. However, if you eat significantly more than this and you are counting calories to lose weight, then you may benefit from using low-fat dairy products.

SHOULD I CHOOSE LOW-FAT DAIRY PRODUCTS?

Low-fat dairy products can be a useful way of reducing your fat and calorie intake, whilst still obtaining the protein and calcium your body needs. Semi-skimmed milk roughly halves the fat content of whole milk and retains some of the flavour. Skimmed milk has most of the fat removed, but as a consequence it has little taste; the choice is yours. Low-fat yoghurts are now so universal it is actually harder to find a full fat version in the supermarket.

One word of caution here: it is common for manufacturers to add sugar or artificial sweeteners to low fat yoghurts to make them palatable, so always check the label. Most cheeses contain 70 – 75% of their calories in fat, which is very high, so choosing a lower fat alternative makes a significant difference. A typical cottage cheese has around 17% fat calories, but the taste and texture is not for everyone. A 'light' cream cheese typically has 40 – 45% fat, which is still high, but a significant overall saving. So if you choose the naturally higher fat option, be aware of your portion size.

WHAT ABOUT LACTOSE INTOLERANCE?

Lactose is a type of sugar found in milk. Virtually all children are able to tolerate lactose well, but as children grow and mature some cease producing the enzyme lactase, which is necessary to digest lactose. They then become lactose intolerant and suffer with gastrointestinal problems, like wind and diarrhoea, if they drink milk.

If you are lactose intolerant and must avoid dairy foods then it is important to have other foods in your diet that are also high in calcium. Examples include green leafy vegetables, such as broccoli and cabbage, soya beans and tofu (soya bean curd), soya drinks with added calcium, nuts, bread and anything made with fortified flour (which has calcium added to it) and fish where you eat the bones, such as sardines and pilchards (www.nhs.uk 2012).

SHOULD I USE PROBIOTICS?

Probiotics are fermented foods such as natural yoghurt or yoghurt-based drinks containing live cultures of 'friendly' bacteria. In principle, if you have enough of these products, the friendly bacteria become established in your large intestine, thus displacing and preventing more harmful bacteria or fungal infections from proliferating and causing ill health. Whether this works in practice is the subject of on-going research. Probiotics come under the heading of 'worth a try', especially if you have been on antibiotics for any reason. However, they are expensive, so if you notice no difference to your health then you are probably wasting your money.

8

HEALTHY FATS

We should aim to eat 2 to 3 portions per day.

Examples of portions include: 2 teaspoons of olive oil, oily fish (size of a deck of cards), ½ an avocado, 2 tablespoons of nuts or seeds.

Healthy fats play an essential part of any diet, with many important functions:

- Fats provide energy in a compact, easily digestible form.
- Fats are important for taste, texture and flavour of foods. A diet entirely devoid of fats is extremely bland and unpalatable.
- Fats are integral to cell membranes and are important for growth and repair of body tissues.
- Fats are a major constituent of brain tissue and insulation of nerves.
- Fats and oils contain the fat soluble vitamins A, D, E and K.
- Omega 3 and omega 6 essential fatty acids (EFAs) are vital for a wide range of functions.
- Body fat offers insulation and protection, and it is a store of energy that we can call on when the energy in our daily diet is not sufficient.
- Body fat is particularly important in women for production and regulation of hormones.

This is quite a list, so it is not surprising that, if you follow a very low-fat diet, you may experience ill health and suffer from, amongst other things, poor skin and hair condition, reduced vitamin status and hormonal deficiencies. Fats are vital, but they have to be healthy fats and they have to be eaten in the right quantity.

HOW CAN I TELL HEALTHY FATS FROM UNHEALTHY FATS?

Fats that are mainly liquid at room temperature are classified as unsaturated. Examples include sunflower oil and olive oil, and the oils found in nuts, seeds and oily fish like mackerel or salmon. Unsaturated fats are therefore mainly vegetable oils and fish oils. Unsaturated fats are generally classified as 'good' fats because some have a beneficial effect on your blood cholesterol level and they also contain good levels of omega 3 and omega 6 EFAs. Unsaturated fats can be further subdivided into 'monounsaturated' and 'polyunsaturated', but the distinctions start to get too complicated for our purposes.

Fats that are mainly solid at room temperature are classified as saturated. Examples include butter, lard, cheese, suet and fat on meat such as bacon or steak. Saturated fats are usually animal fats, although palm oil and coconut oil are exceptions to this rule. Pizza and cheese are the biggest food sources of saturated fat in the diet, and other dairy products and meat products are also major contributors (www.hsph.harvard.edu 2012).

Saturated fats are generally classified as 'bad' fats because some have a harmful effect on your blood cholesterol level.

SHOULD WE SIMPLY REPLACE SATURATED FATS FOR UNSATURATED FATS?

As with all the food groups, fats should be present in your diet in their most natural form. For example, saturated fat intrinsically present in meat or unsaturated fat in nuts and seeds. It would not be advisable to increase your consumption of highly processed and refined unsaturated liquid oils.

HOW DO FATS AFFECT BLOOD CHOLESTEROL AND HEART DISEASE?

Blood cholesterol level is considered to be a major indicator of developing heart disease and you will probably have had your cholesterol measured by your doctor as part of a regular health check.

The term 'blood cholesterol level' is commonly used, but not really correct. Rather it is the *carriers* of cholesterol in the blood that are being measured, and these are called lipoproteins. Increased levels of low-density lipoproteins (LDLs) in particular are linked with fatty deposits clogging the insides of arteries, eventually leading to a blockage. If a blockage happens to build up in the vital coronary arteries that supply the heart with blood, then angina or even a heart attack can result. This is the concern with some saturated fats: they are the ones that increase your LDLs, encouraging clogging of the arteries, leading to heart disease. Some unsaturated fats don't seem to increase LDLs; in fact, they may actually reduce levels.

At this point you may be thinking, 'Why don't I only eat unsaturated, good fats and eliminate all saturated, bad fats from my diet?'

Although this is an obvious conclusion, this is not actually possible because all foods contain a mix of both types of fat. Even 'good' fats in fish, nuts or olive oil contain *some* saturated fat, though they are much lower than cheese or meat. Similarly, saturated fats like cheese, butter or lard all contain some unsaturated fat too. The categorisation in the first place is made based on which type of fat is the higher percentage.

Realistic practical advice is not to try to eliminate, but to shift your *balance* of fats from cheese, meat and dairy to fish, nuts and good quality, unrefined oils. And when you do eat animal fats, choose better quality products, not processed ones.

WHICH IS HEALTHIER: BUTTER OR MARGARINE?

From the preceding argument, it should be clear that butter, with a high saturated fat content (around 66%) is an unhealthy choice compared to margarine (more commonly called a 'spread') with a much lower saturated fat (around 27%). In addition, many brands of margarine will offer:

- a 'light' option that has reduced total fat content and roughly halves the calories
- a 'cholesterol lowering' option containing plant sterols. These are chemicals found naturally in vegetable oils, fruits and vegetables that reduce the amount of cholesterol absorbed by your gut, hence reducing levels of LDL (bad) cholesterol in your blood
- an 'omega 3' option with added omega 3 essential fatty acids.

Yet even with all these arguments, there are still some positive points for butter. It certainly tastes better, no question. It is more stable at high temperatures and therefore more suitable for cooking. Butter naturally supplies significant amounts of omega 3 EFA, and it has minimal processing compared to spreads and therefore contains no harmful 'trans' fats (see next section).

WHAT ARE OMEGA 3 AND OMEGA 6 EFAS?

Omega 3 and 6 EFAs are specific types of fat found predominantly in unsaturated oils from fish, seeds and nuts.

An adequate intake of omega 3 EFAs reduces blood clotting, having the effect of 'thinning the blood' and helping to lower blood pressure. This in turn reduces your chances of getting a blocked artery or suffering from a heart attack. There are also anti-inflammatory effects which can be beneficial to your joints, and there may be an association between dietary omega 3 and alleviating depression.

Omega 6 EFAs are vital for healthy structure and functioning of cell membranes and particularly important for healthy skin. They may also reduce LDL (bad) cholesterol levels.

A typical diet in today's developed countries is plentiful in omega 6 because of widespread use of vegetable oils. In contrast, omega 3 consumption is more limited and authorities agree that we would benefit from a higher intake. The most effective way to do this is to include 2 to 3 portions of oily fish, like mackerel or salmon, in the diet each week. If you don't like the taste of oily fish, or your budget and culinary skills won't stretch to having 2 to 3 servings per week, then there are other options.

Seeds and nuts also contain significant quantities of omega 3, but in the less potent 'short chain' form found in vegetable sources. Many products like spreads, yoghurts, bread and eggs now have omega 3 added as part of the production process (extra omega 3 in eggs comes from mixing flax and hemp seeds into the chicken feed). And if none of this tempts you, then fish oil supplements such as traditional cod liver oil can be a convenient alternative. If you find the fish flavour too unpleasant then capsules with a tasteless coating are now widely available.

NOTE: Large doses of omega 3 EFAs can have a significant effect on blood clotting times. Anyone already taking blood thinning medication should consult their doctor before using fish oil supplements.

A few key points to remember from this section:

- Limit your total portions of healthy fats to 2 to 3 per day.
- Shift your *balance* of fats from cheese, meat and dairy products to

fish, nuts and good quality, unrefined oils to reduce your intake of saturated fats and increase your intake of unsaturated fats.

- Regularly eat fats that are a good source of omega 3 and 6 EFAs. Oily fish like salmon and mackerel are particularly good for omega 3.

9

UNHEATHY FATS AND REFINED SUGAR

We should aim to eat only 0 to 1 portion per day.

Examples of portions include: 1 biscuit, 1 slice of cake, 1 can of soft drink, 25g (1oz) bag of crisps, 1 small bowl of chocolate pudding, 125ml glass fruit juice or smoothie (if you have more than 1 per day).

The smallest segment of the food plate is for foods high in unhealthy fats and refined sugar. We should aim to eat them in only small quantities, or not at all.

Foods high in unhealthy fats include: Lard, cream, cheese, mayonnaise, meat, pies, chips and crisps.

Foods high in refined sugar include: Jam, marmalade, sugar in tea and coffee, and fruit juices (if you have more than 1 portion per day). Cans of soft drink are a major source of refined sugar in the average diet.

Foods high in both unhealthy fats and refined sugar include: Cakes, doughnuts, flapjacks, muffins, pastries, biscuits, ice cream and chocolate. These are particularly hard for us to resist.

Many of these are highly processed, refined products that are cleverly marketed. This combination of factors makes them hard for us to resist. Foods that contain a combination of fat and sugar or fat and salt are particularly appealing to our taste buds. They feed our natural cravings and there is good evidence that they stimulate the same areas of the brain as addictive drugs.

We are advised to eat these foods sparingly because they are very high in calories that are easy to digest (very 'fattening') but often low in vitamins, minerals and fibre. However, we find it hard to follow this advice because they are so tasty and so widely available. No wonder it is so easy to gain weight. Some planning and self-discipline is called for.

PROCESSING, HYDROGENATION AND 'TRANS' FATS

Processing of fats in particular can have health implications. More than 100 years ago, food manufacturers worked out how to make vegetable oils more solid or spreadable by a factory process called 'hydrogenation'. This is useful to the manufacturer because vegetable oils are inexpensive compared to animal fats, so products like cakes and biscuits can be made more cheaply. Hydrogenation also increases the stability of the fat, improving the shelf life of the product in the supermarket.

However, the hydrogenation process results in some harmful 'trans' fats being present in the food. Trans fats have just a slightly different molecular arrangement from unprocessed fats, but this is enough for your body to treat them in a different way, leading to increased LDL (bad) cholesterol and possibly a number of other health consequences. You are well advised to eliminate trans fats from your diet.

Food products that may contain trans fats are cakes, biscuits, ready meals, chocolate, chips, crisps and spreads. A good rule is to be cautious with any highly processed products, but it is hard to tell for certain. The best way to tell is to look for 'hydrogenated vegetable fat' or similar on the list of ingredients. Trans fats are sometimes, but not always, identified specifically on the nutrition label.

Governments and food producers have long been aware of the problems with trans fats and, to a large extent, have changed laws and manufacturing processes to reduce them to negligible levels. Most premium brand margarines and spreads sold today contain only tiny amounts, but cheaper brands can still be a concern. Check the label to be sure.

WHAT ABOUT ARTIFICIAL SWEETENERS?

Artificial sweeteners are commonly used in diet soft drinks. There are also sweeteners that can be used in coffee and tea, or sugar substitutes to sprinkle on your breakfast cereal. These products can certainly be useful to cut down sugar and calorie intake whilst still satisfying a sweet tooth. Just be aware that there is some concern as to whether they interfere with natural appetite control. The theory is that your body *expects* calories from the sweetness it tastes, but actually *receives* none. The brain then recalibrates your appetite, asking for more sweet food until it gets the calories it expects. A sensible approach is to use artificially sweetened products in moderation.

10

WHAT TO DRINK

A healthy guideline is to drink about 1 to 1.5 litres (6 to 8 glasses) of plain water each day, enough to prevent thirst.

Your body naturally loses fluid each day through natural processes and functions. Most fluid is lost as:

- Sweat
- Urine
- Faeces
- Water vapour in breath

There may be other less significant fluid loss from tears, bleeding, mucus, etc. (you can complete this particular list yourself).

On a typical day these daily losses total about 2 to 2.5 litres, so it follows that you need to replace this quantity of fluid to remain hydrated. Of course, factors such as larger body size, hot weather, exercise or illness can increase this fluid loss, so consider 2 to 2.5 litres as a baseline loss. You may lose considerably more.

However, note that food itself contains water, so even if you drank nothing in a day you would still obtain about 1 litre of fluid just from eating; more if you consume high quantities of fruit and vegetables. Hence we arrive at the general guideline of drinking 1 to 1.5 litres (about 6 to 8 glasses) of plain water each day.

Drinking more water than you need has no additional benefits. You will simply excrete it as urine a while later and it does no harm. Be aware that there are *extreme* circumstances usually associated with illness or endurance races, where too much water can dilute the sodium in the blood causing a serious condition called hyponatraemia. Consult a dietician if you have any concerns.

If you don't like the idea of drinking just plain water, remember that most drinks consist mainly of water and, contrary to received wisdom, will rehydrate to some extent. This includes tea, coffee, fizzy drinks, beer, milk and fruit juice. They may not be *ideal* because of their caffeine, sugar and alcohol content, but they do all contribute to fluid intake and can keep you hydrated.

HOW CAN I TELL IF I AM FULLY HYDRATED?

Keeping hydrated is important for most bodily functions including circulation, cell metabolism, digestion, temperature regulation and elimination of waste. If you become dehydrated, then it will affect the efficiency of all these processes. Your body will detect mild dehydration and this will make you feel thirsty, which will prompt you to have a drink and rehydrate. If you are losing larger volumes of fluid as sweat because of exercise or humidity, you will feel thirstier and drink more – a simple feedback loop that has served humans well for thousands of years.

If you don't drink and dehydration becomes more severe, it starts to affect blood circulation, saliva production and urine volume. You will notice symptoms such as headache, nausea, dry mouth and darker coloured urine (clear or pale 'straw coloured' urine is a reliable indicator of hydration). But usually you will feel thirsty and drink long before these symptoms appear. Severe dehydration is more commonly the result of illness, excessive alcohol consumption, or extreme circumstances when no water is available.

So if you don't feel thirsty and your urine colour is clear or pale yellow, you can be confident you are fully hydrated (note: if your urine is bright yellow after taking a vitamin supplement, don't worry, it's a side effect of vitamin B_2, not dehydration).

CAN SPORTS DRINKS HELP ME TO REHYDRATE?

Sports drinks labelled as 'isotonic' or 'hypotonic' may be able to hydrate you a little faster than water. This is because they contain small amounts of sugars and salts (electrolytes) that help absorption of the water from the stomach into your blood and cells. The sugar content also supplies some energy if you are training. However, it is debatable as to whether the small advantage they give is significant for most exercise sessions unless they last longer than one hour.

Some sports drinks come under the heading of 'energy drinks' because of their high sugar content. Although they do supply energy, the greater sugar content slows absorption of fluid from your stomach and their ability to rehydrate you quickly is reduced. Most energy drinks contain significant amounts of caffeine.

WHAT ABOUT CAFFEINE DRINKS?

Drinks such as coffee, tea and cola all contain caffeine. Caffeine is a stimulant drug that occurs in the seeds (e.g. coffee beans) and leaves (e.g. tea leaves) of some plants. It is also added to cola and most energy drinks. Caffeine acts on our central nervous system, making us more alert and more energetic and improving athletic performance, so it is not surprising that most of us like to have our daily 'fix'. Along with alcohol, caffeine is the most widely consumed drug in the world.

Individual tolerance to caffeine varies widely. Some people will feel little effect, whereas others experience sleep disorders and anxiety. Your own experience makes you the best judge here. However, the stimulant benefits from caffeine also have a downside.

Caffeine is a known diuretic. In other words, caffeine stimulates increased urine production, which may lead to dehydration. However, the significance of this is debatable. Caffeine drinks like coffee, tea or cola contribute to fluid intake because they are mostly water anyway, and this intake typically exceeds the fluid loss from the diuretic effect. Also, regular consumers of caffeine seem to develop a tolerance to its effects, making fluid loss virtually negligible.

Like any stimulant drug, a caffeine dependency can develop and withdrawal can be hard. People who stop taking in caffeine typically experience headache, fatigue, lack of concentration and lethargy. If you have a few days with nothing important to deal with, it can be revealing to try going 'cold turkey' and find out how dependent you might have become.

Excessive caffeine intake is, along with many other things, associated with an increased risk of heart disease.

So the sensible advice with caffeine drinks is to have them regularly in moderation or not at all. If you regularly drink coffee, tea or cola, 2 to 3 a day is acceptable, and they will contribute some useful fluid to keep you hydrated (though not as much as if you drank plain water). Alternatively, decaffeinated coffees and teas are widely available.

SHOULD I DRINK ALCOHOL?

There is absolutely no need for humans to drink alcohol. It serves no nutritional purpose, it is toxic and if you drink enough alcohol it can kill you. In the short term, alcohol is a diuretic and will dehydrate the body. Compare the symptoms of dehydration (headache, nausea, dry mouth, etc.) to those of a hangover and you find they are very similar. Alcoholic drinks are also high in calories and contribute significantly to gaining body fat. In addition, there are a whole range of other associated problems:

- Decreased sexual performance, especially for men
- Increased risk of cancer of the throat, oesophagus or larynx
- Increased risk of breast cancer in women
- Increased risk of stroke, heart disease and heart attack
- High blood pressure
- Liver disease such as cirrhosis
- Pancreatitis
- Reduced fertility

Having said all this, alcohol in moderation can actually have some positive health benefits. It can help people to cope with stress, relax, unwind and be more sociable, there is a small but noticeable blood thinning effect, and certain drinks like red wine, beer and stout contain vitamins, minerals and antioxidants.

So if a daily glass of wine or beer is important to you it isn't essential to give it up. Instead, the key phrase here is *in moderation.*

WHAT IS A MODERATE ALCOHOL INTAKE?

The easiest way to check that you are keeping to a moderate intake is to stay within your 'lower risk guidelines' per day.

Women should not exceed 2 to 3 units per day. This is roughly equivalent to a 175ml glass of wine.

Men should not exceed 3 to 4 units per day. This is roughly equivalent to a strong pint of beer, lager or cider.
(www.nhs.uk 2012).

There are now various websites and phone apps to help you check how many units you are drinking. The men's guideline is higher than the women's simply because of a larger average body size. Alcohol affects each individual differently depending on circumstances, amount of food in the stomach (which slows absorption) and even genetics. Note also that staying within the lower risk guidelines does not guarantee you are legally safe to drive.

11

REDUCING SALT INTAKE

If you would like to avoid having high blood pressure (hypertension), one dietary change you should make is to eat less salt. This has been shown to give modest reductions in blood pressure for most people, which in turn will decrease your risk of health problems such as heart disease and stroke.

The sodium in salt (sodium chloride) is important for fluid balance within your body. If you eat too much salt your body tends to retain more water, which leads to an increased blood pressure. The problem is that salt is a common ingredient in foods. It is a traditional preservative used in canned products, and we seem to crave the flavour and taste. Much of the salt we eat is already in foods such as bread, breakfast cereal and ready meals.
Current guidelines suggest we should eat just 6g of salt per day, which is about a teaspoon. But unless you are particularly careful about your intake already, you are likely to be eating double that amount, at around 11g per day (www.nhs.uk 2012).

HOW CAN I CUT MY SALT INTAKE?

A few simple steps can help you to reduce your salt intake.

Firstly, don't add salt when cooking, or if it is essential to the recipe, keep it to a minimum. Next, don't add extra salt to your food at the table. If you have developed a taste for salt and find this hard, then cut down gradually over a number of weeks. If you really can't kick the habit of adding salt to your food, one further option is to use a low sodium alternative that has the same taste, but only one third of the sodium.

Lastly, avoid foods that are obviously high in salt, such as anchovies, bacon, cheese, crisps, ham, olives, pickles, salami, salted nuts, salt fish, smoked meat and fish, soya sauce, stock cubes and yeast extract. Foods containing monosodium glutamate (MSG), a flavour enhancer used in savoury dishes, should also be avoided.

These simple measures will make a significant difference to your salt intake. However, to really cut down, use the nutrition labels on food packaging. Salt is in so many everyday foods where you might not expect it. By reading the labels you can select lower salt options reliably and stay within the 6g per day limit.

12

SHOPPING, COOKING AND EATING OUT

So far we have outlined the key principles of healthy eating, but they are no use unless you can apply them easily on a daily basis – which brings us on to shopping, food preparation and eating out.

WHAT DO I LOOK FOR WHEN SHOPPING?

Food manufacturers and supermarkets are very good at selling us products that are not necessarily healthy, so when you go shopping you need to be prepared. Have a list based around balanced meals and whole foods and then apply a little discipline to stick to your list. Remember, what you buy will fill your refrigerator for the next week and forms the basis of what you will eat.

Healthy foods actually *look* like proper food. You can tell they came from something that was once living: fruit, veg, cereal grains, nuts, fish, meat and poultry. They are fresh (or possibly frozen) and naturally coloured. Dieticians use the phrase 'good food goes off quickly' – emphasising the importance of freshness and the lack of processing and preservatives. In contrast, unhealthy foods look processed, packaged and artificial. They are likely to be high in processed fats and refined sugars, and they probably contain salt, trans-fats, chemical preservatives, colourings and flavourings to make them more appealing and to prolong shelf life.

Most supermarkets follow a similar floor plan, with the freshest food kept on the shelves closest to their storerooms, because they have to restock them regularly throughout the day. You can check next time you are there.

Soon after the entrance you will encounter fresh produce – fruit and vegetables. Then if you stay to the perimeter shelves, you will find fresh fish, meat and poultry, dairy, eggs, usually finishing with the bakery and frozen foods just before the checkout. Frozen vegetables are good in terms of freshness because of the speed with which they are frozen and preserved following harvesting. Items with an extended shelf life, such as tinned foods, breakfast cereals, biscuits, sugary drinks, sweets and snacks tend to be in the middle of the supermarket because they need restocking less frequently.

So an easy rule when shopping is to prioritise fresh food from around the outer shelves and counters of the supermarket. Better still, if you have the time, buy your food from a local farmers' market.

HOW DO I USE FOOD LABELS?

Food labels can be useful for checking specific details. For example, the list of ingredients will tell you if the product contains hydrogenated fats, added sugar or salt. If you have an allergy to a particular food then you can check the ingredients to make sure you don't eat that food by mistake. Staple foods such as wheat, eggs and milk are in many products where you might not expect them.

The nutrition label can be used to check exact amounts of energy, fats, carbs and proteins in the product and whether it supplies significant amounts of calcium, salt, fibre, etc. Other labelling codes use a 'traffic light' colour system or a 'guideline daily amount' (GDA) system that can be useful for comparing the calories, total fat, saturated fat, sugar and salt content of different products. There could also be other helpful information such as the GI of the food, or specific health claims such as 'can help to lower cholesterol'.

All of this information can be useful to help you select healthier options when shopping. However, if you feel overwhelmed with the mass of figures, and don't want to carry a reference book and calculator around the store with you, then don't worry – it's not essential. Just stick to the rules about buying fresh whole foods and eating according to the food plate and the figures will take care of themselves.

WHAT ARE THE HEALTHIEST COOKING METHODS?

Once you have stocked your cupboards and refrigerator with healthy foods, a little thought needs to be devoted to how you prepare them. For example, it is wise to choose a cooking method that does not add unnecessary fat. Grilling meat with just a drizzle of olive oil is a more sensible choice than deep frying or roasting which results in a much higher fat content. Deep fried foods are a known source of damaging free radicals, caused by the frying oil being oxidised when it is repeatedly heated at a high temperature. If you do occasionally fry food it is actually best to use a solid, saturated animal fat like butter or lard because they are much more stable at high temperatures and less likely to oxidise compared to unsaturated oils.

The cooking method you choose is also important for preserving the vitamins, minerals and phytochemical content of the food. Contrary to popular belief, eating all raw vegetables is not necessarily the healthiest choice. Boiling vegetables for a long time will certainly destroy some of the vitamin C content because it is unstable and easily degraded through exposure to heat. But other vitamins, such as beta carotene (which your body converts into vitamin A) can actually be made more accessible from cooking. A sensible compromise is to lightly steam or stir fry vegetables. If you boil veg as part of a meal, use the water to make a stock or gravy. Microwave cooking is actually quite good for preserving vitamin and mineral content of foods. However, this should not be used as an excuse to eat lots of microwave ready meals.

You should wash fruit and veg thoroughly before eating them. Sometimes peeling is recommended (www.nhs.uk 2012). This ensures they are safe to eat by reducing the chances of bacterial infection or food poisoning. It may also be important to wash fruit and veg because of the pesticide residues. However, in most cases the presence of the residues found would be unlikely to have any effect on your health (www.pesticides.gov.uk 2012)

WHAT ABOUT EATING OUT AND TAKEAWAYS?

It can be hard to follow a healthy eating plan when eating out or ordering a takeaway. But there are some simple rules you can follow to help:

- At the restaurant, have two courses, not three. This could be a starter then a main, but miss out dessert. Or, alternatively, skip the starter if you particularly look forward to dessert.
- Order a side salad with the main course. This is a great way to help meet your veg intake.
- Avoid dishes that are deep fried.
- If someone asks, 'Do you want cheese with that?' just say no.
- Avoid creamy sauces on your steak or pasta dishes, or mayonnaise on your sandwich.
- At the pizzeria, choose a traditional Italian-base pizza. This has much less fat than a deep pan or stuffed crust version.
- If the dish is served with a choice of fried, boiled or mashed potatoes, avoid the fried option to help reduce fat.

And finally, remember that eating out should be a pleasurable, sociable occasion. Don't become a food bore. If you lapse a little it doesn't matter. Just get back on track the next day.

13

EFFECTIVE WEIGHT MANAGEMENT

Finally we will look at how to manage weight in the long term without resorting to the latest trendy idea or diet. There is no need for a system, secret or fad when it comes to losing fat and maintaining a healthy body weight. On the contrary, it is just a matter of following the principles we have already discussed in the previous sections.

WHAT IS A HEALTHY BODY WEIGHT?

Aside from looking in the mirror, you can use body mass index (BMI) to check if you are a healthy weight. The calculation is as follows:

BMI = weight (kg) ÷ height² (m)

For example, if you weigh 87kg and your height is 1.81m, your BMI is:

87 ÷ (1.81 x 1.81) = 87 ÷ 3.276 = <u>26.5</u>

Then compare the figure to the chart below:

BMI	Category
Less than 19	Underweight
19 - 25	Healthy weight
25 - 29	Overweight
More than 30	Obese

So a BMI of 26.5 falls in the 'overweight' category. If you lost 7kg (roughly one stone) then the BMI would reduce to 24.4 and be in the 'healthy' category, leading to decreased risk of high blood pressure, heart disease, non-insulin dependent diabetes and arthritis in your knees and hips as you get older.

However, Central YMCA and the All Party Parliamentary Group (APPG) on Body Image recently called for Body Mass Index to be revised. The measure was developed in the 1830s to compare large swathes of populations and while it is a useful indicator at epidemiological levels, the APPG argues that it is a blunt and inaccurate measure of someone's health. For example, BMI says nothing about body composition, such as level of muscularity or bone density. It also doesn't give an indication of where fat is distributed within the body i.e. visceral or subcutaneous.

The APPG concluded that BMI should be reviewed, and potentially revised to take account of differences in genders, age groups and ethnicities. It also believes that BMI should be used in collaboration with other health indicators, such as waist circumference or measure of subjective wellbeing, to more accurately indicate a person's overall health.

HOW CAN I START TO LOSE WEIGHT GRADUALLY?

We know from the energy balance equations that, to maintain weight, calories eaten must equal calories expended, not necessarily exactly every day, but over the long term this needs to be the case.

To lose weight it follows that we need to create an energy deficit, with less being eaten than is being expended. But if this energy deficit is too severe (i.e. if you go on a diet) then there are many negative health consequences. Moreover, a severe deficit is not sustainable. Instead, your aim should be a modest reduction in calories, giving steady weight loss, but avoiding all the problems of dieting and then relapsing.

WHAT IS THE EASIEST WAY TO REDUCE CALORIE INTAKE?

A modest reduction in calories can be easily achieved using the following measures:

- Use portion control. Become familiar with portion sizes and stick to the food plate as a guide to how many portions should be eaten.
- Use a smaller dinner plate. A simple way to implement portion control is to replace the large 30cm (12 inch) dinner plates in your

cupboard with smaller 23cm (9 inch) ones. This measure has been shown to reduce the quantity of food prepared and served, and therefore reduce how much we eat on a daily basis.

- Limit your intake of foods high in processed fats and sugars. This is where a majority of excess calories are consumed. If you don't cut your intake of these 'junk' foods it is hard to stick to your calorie count for the day. Have them as the occasional treat.

Reading this you will probably argue, with some justification, that removing high fat and sugar foods will make you feel hungry all the time. But there are several steps you can take to help to control your appetite.

HOW CAN I CONTROL MY APPETITE?

Much has been discovered recently about what controls our appetite and what makes us hungry. The results are surprisingly complex, with factors such as habit, emotions, stomach fullness, blood sugar levels and hunger hormones all playing a part. Without delving too deeply into the science, the following measures all help you to control your appetite and calorie intake:

- Eat 5 to 6 times per day. Have a structured meal plan with breakfast, lunch, dinner and two or three healthy snacks in between. In particular, don't miss breakfast. Missing meals triggers various hunger hormones which in turn cause you to crave high fat and sugar calories at the next meal.
- Eat some protein at each meal. Adequate protein seems to suppress hunger and is another key to controlling appetite.
- Choose unrefined complex carbohydrates. They are relatively bulky foods that help to fill the stomach, and they are also low GI which helps to keep you feeling fuller for longer.
- Eat at least 5 a day of fruit and vegetables for the same reasons.
- Take a normal meal and blend it with some water to make a soup. This blending into a soup makes the same meal slower to digest. It stays in the stomach, keeping it distended for longer. This leaves you feeling fuller for longer and less likely to snack before your next meal time.
- Drink some water before each meal. You may have heard the idea that the body can 'mistake hunger for thirst' and that if you feel hungry, drink a glass of water and your hunger will subside. Whilst there is little evidence for this specific claim, it does seem that drinking a glass of water (500ml) before meals reduces subsequent calorie consumption in that meal. This is not a massive effect, but

the technique may help as part of an overall weight loss plan.

That's it. No carb curfew, no blood group analysis, no rotation of food groups or protein days followed by carb days. Just guidelines based on sound nutrition principles that are sustainable in the long term.

Of course the other key part of weight control is increasing activity and exercise; the 'energy out' side of the equation. But for now that is enough healthy advice to get you started. The exercise part will have to wait for another day.

BIBLIOGRAPHY AND WEBSITES OF INTEREST

www.choosemyplate.gov (2012).
www.dh.gov.uk (2012).
www.diabetes.org.uk (2012).
www.earlybirddiabetes.org (2012).
www.hsph.harvard.edu (2012).
www.nhs.uk (2012).
www.pesticides.gov.uk (2012).

Bean, A. (2003). *The Complete Guide to Sports Nutrition*. London: A & C Black.
Foster, R., & Kreitzman, L. (2005). *Rhythms of Life. The Biological Clocks that Control the Daily Lives of Every Living Thing*. London: Profile Books Ltd.

THE CENTRAL YMCA GUIDES SERIES

Happy and Healthy: A collection of trustworthy advice on health, fitness and wellbeing topics

UK
http://www.centralymcaguides.com/hhct2

US
http://www.centralymcaguides.com/hhct

The Scientific Approach to Exercise for Fat Loss: How to get in shape and shed unwanted fat by using healthy and scientifically proven techniques

UK
http://www.centralymcaguides.com/sael2

US
http://www.centralymcaguides.com/sael

The Need to Know Guide to Nutrition for Exercise: How your food and drink can help you to achieve your workout goals

UK
http://www.centralymcaguides.com/ngne2

US
http://www.centralymcaguides.com/ngne

The Need to Know Guide to Nutrition and Healthy Eating: The perfect starter to eating well or how to eat the right foods, stay in shape and stick to a healthy diet

UK
http://www.centralymcaguides.com/gnhe2

US http://www.centralymcaguides.com/gnhe

Tri Harder - The A to Z of Triathlon for Improvers: The triathlon competitors' guide to training and improving your running, cycling and swimming times

UK
http://www.centralymcaguides.com/thtc2

US http://www.centralymcaguides.com/thtc

20 Full Body Training Programmes for Exercise Lovers: An essential guide to boosting your general fitness, strength, power and endurance

UK http://www.centralymcaguides.com/tpel2

US http://www.centralymcaguides.com/tpel

Run, Jump, Climb, Crawl: The essential training guide for obstacle racing enthusiasts, or how to get fit, stay safe and prepare for the toughest mud runs on the planet

UK
http://www.centralymcaguides.com/rjc2

US
http://www.centralymcaguides.com/rjc

Gardening for Health: The Need to Know Guide to the Health Benefits of Horticulture

UK
http://www.centralymcaguides.com/gfhh2

US
http://www.centralymcaguides.com/gfhh

New Baby, New You: The Need to Know Guide to Postnatal Health and Happiness - How to return to exercise and get back in shape after giving birth

UK
http://www.centralymcaguides.com/nbny2

US
http://www.centralymcaguides.com/nbny

The Need to Know Guide to Life with a Toddler and a Newborn: How to prepare for and cope with the day to day challenge of raising two young children

UK
http://www.centralymcaguides.com/ngtn2

US
http://www.centralymcaguides.com/ngtn

50 Games for Active Toddlers: Quick everyday hints and tips to keep toddlers active, healthy and occupied

UK
http://www.centralymcaguides.com/50uk

US
http://www.centralymcaguides.com/50us

Exercise and Nutrition 3 Book Bundle

UK
http://www.centralymcaguides.com/enb2

US
http://www.centralymcaguides.com/enb

Obstacle Racing Preparation 3 Book Bundle

UK
http://www.centralymcaguides.com/orpb2

US
http://www.centralymcaguides.com/orpb

Nutrition and Fat Loss 3 Book Bundle

UK
http://www.centralymcaguides.com/nflb2

US
http://www.centralymcaguides.com/nflb

Mums' Health 3 Book Bundle

UK
http://www.centralymcaguides.com/mhb2

US
http://www.centralymcaguides.com/mhb

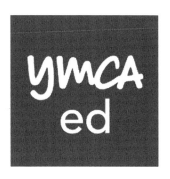

Discover more books and ebooks of interest to you and find out about the range of work we do at the forefront of health, fitness and wellbeing.

www.centralymcaguides.com

Printed in Great Britain
by Amazon